Disclaimer

Remember to never use any essential oils without first consulting with a doctor. If you have skin allergies talk to your dermatologist before using any new product on your skin. The author of this book is not a medical doctor and cannot be held liable for negative reactions to these products. Any use of these recipes is strictly at your own risk. Use with caution.

To begin...

Sometimes the best way to know how you will react to certain bath salts, is to begin with a plain bath, using no salts or other ingredients in the water, and compare that bath to a plain salt bath. If you had a good experience with just taking a water bath, you will have something to compare the plain salt bath to. Starting slow has no shame in it, just being cautious is a wonderful way to express to your mind, body, and spirit, that you are changing your habits to better suit them and not the world around you. Your first step is to make sure you have a great experience using all of these recipes, and giving yourself a moment to figure out how these baths will work for you.

Blessings.

To begin...

1 Cup Epsom Salt

1 Tablespoon Rose or Orange water

Combine ingredients. Do not add color or oils, perfumes, or other scented products.

Makes enough for two baths.

words and such...

Mind:

Body:

Soul:

Peace....

Even on our busiest days it is best to just be still for a moment and know you are loved and wanted. Baths are a great way of letting the world know you are busy taking care of you. Ironically, this time really does belong to you since most people will not bother you in the bath. This is your time for peace. Peace of mind, peace of heart, peace of soul. Getting into a warm bath, full of warm scents, will carry you through those hours that are demanded of you to give to others. While you are expected to do it all, you are expected to be still as well, this should be done with an open heart, since it's where you draw your strength from.

Peace...

1 cup Epsom salt

20 drops Cinnamon Oil

20 drops Sandalwood Oil

1 tablespoon Jasmine Water

Combine all ingredients in a small bowl.

Store in clear glass bottles.

Add roughly 1/4 of mix to running water in bath.

Makes enough for two baths

words and such...

Mind:

Body:

Soul:

Prepare...

With days ahead that require your thoughts and actions in full swing with the events to come, try to take a moment and settle into a mind clearing state so that you may better handle the stressful events in the near future. These events can be a full calendar for the week, projects for an up and coming holiday or just a dinner party for your friends. Whatever the occasion may be, being prepared is your best defense against any bumps you may encounter on that road. There is always some per-preparations to do before you get to the actual process of getting things done, and this bath time is it. By preparing yourself before the event planning, you have a upper hand on all of the little things that like to pop up when you are busy dealing with the details. There is nothing more important then making sure you are ready for the tasks ahead, so take some time and prepare yourself first.

Prepare...

1 cup Epsom salt

1/2 teaspoon Cedarwood Oil

1/2 teaspoon Pachouli Oil

Combine all ingredients in a small bowl.

Store in clear glass bottles.

Add roughly 1/4 of mix to running water in bath.

Enough to make two baths

words and such...

Mind:

Body:

Soul:

Joy...

For those days and nights that you just cannot contain yourself within four walls, this bath salt is just for that. When you are ready to paint the town red, so to speak, take a warm bath with this bath salt recipe and allow yourself to have an even better experience. There is no rule that says you cannot enjoy life sometimes and just have fun, and this blend is just for those occasions. Even if you plan to spend a night in with friends or loved family, cherish them a little more because you took some time to be joyful just for you. No matter what the need for joy may be, you can add more whenever you are ready.

Joy...

1/2 cup dead sea salt

10 drops Ylang Ylang oil

Combine all ingredients in a small bowl.

Store in clear glass bottles.

Add roughly 1/4 of mix to running water in bath.

Enough for two baths

words and such...

Mind:

Body:

Soul:

Slow down...

One of the things we usually forget to do is slow down and make time for ourselves. This isn't new to us and we know we need to take a deep breathe in order to see the wonders around us. With life getting closer and closer to the fast track, slowing down sometimes does not seem like a solution to better any situation,or so it goes. When we slow down we see situations for what they are, something we can easily manage and take in stride. We do forget that by slowing down our stresses do not take on a life of their own anymore. Bath salts are a great companion to remind us that we can solve our stresses and still have the energy to follow through with our solutions.

Slow down...

1 cup Epsom salt

10 drops Pine Oil

10 drops Peppermint Oil

Combine all ingredients in a small bowl.

Store in clear glass bottles.

Add roughly 1/4 of mix to running water in bath.

Enough to make two baths

words and such....

Mind:

Body:

Soul:

Harmony...

Living among the hustle and bustle of the city and home lives, harmony is a difficult place to find. While we try to complete daily tasks and plan for future endeavors we take ourselves to the brink of disconnectedness. Harmony must begin with you. Once you open yourself to this, harmony then comes to you. A bath mix has helped me in times of loss of focus, feelings of disconnectedness, and on days I have just felt like I was being left behind. Harmony was what I need most and this bath helped me find it. The need for harmony is for everyone, and everyone needs a few minutes to find that harmony connection.

Harmony...

1 cup Epsom salt

20 drops of Vanilla Oil

20 drops of Ylang Ylang Oil

20 drops of Neroli Oil

1 tablespoon of Rosewater

4 drops of Green food coloring (optional)

Combine all ingredients in a small bowl.

Make sure food coloring is completely absorbed and color is even.

Store in clear glass bottles.

Add roughly 1/4 of the mix into running water in bath.

Enough for two baths

words and such...

Mind:

Body:

Soul:

Eden in my life...

There are days when we want to lose ourselves in perfection. When we want to connect so badly to that which is divine. This bath mix is just for such occasions. The perfection may be a garden that visited once or perhaps many times. Perfection could be a day when the one's you love where close by and laughing. Or maybe even an entire block of time that you have claimed as the best of your life. The need to feel perfection begins with a longing. A wonderment of things that once were, things that began a good feeling, places such as Eden. Though Eden is no longer available to us, blessings are. Good memories are always available and so are blessings.

Eden...

1 cup Epsom salt

30 drops Rosemary Oil

30 drops Citronella Oil

30 drops Lavender Oil

1 Tablespoon Rosewater

4 drops of Blue food coloring (optional)

Combine all ingredients in a small bowl.

Make sure food coloring is completely absorbed and color is even.

Store in clear glass bottles.

Add roughly 1/4 of the mix into running water in bath.

Enough for two baths

words and such...

Mind:

Body:

Soul:

Rejoicing...

Spring is a blessed event. The change from the cold season to the warm. Feeling the sun

on your face again. Hearing the sound of birds, waterfalls, and the warmer wind

through the trees. Such an awakening happens every year, and so it does to people as

well. It is a blessed time for us, and the changes happen in us as well. The bath mix is

for those times when you begin to smell the Jasmine in the air, or asses the garden you

want this summer. Celebrating the rebirth of everything around us. A time to spread

our own wings and fly once again. Enjoy this bath mix whenever you miss the Spring

season or wish to remember Spring season that have already passed.

Rejoicing...

2 cups Epsom salt

30 drops Rose Oil

30 drops Lilac Oil

30 drops Honeysuckle Oil

30 drops Vanilla Oil

30 drops Jasmine Oil

10 drops Rose Oil

10 drops Lavender Oil

Combine all ingredients in a small bowl.

Store in clear glass bottles.

Add roughly 1/4 of mix to running water in bath.

Enough for two baths

words and such...

Mind:

Body:

Soul:

Winter...

Hot cups of coco, warm blankets, soft sweaters, and the fun of shopping. These are all things we do in the winter time. Whether is preparing for the holidays, or just having a quite dinner at home. This time of year is meant for you to be close to those you love and to love them even more. This bath salt is here for use when you want those winter joys you have last just a little bit longer. So before you take out the decorations, put an extra log on the fire, or get your camera ready, use this bath salt to help you feel the festive atmosphere you are about to create. So get yourself ready!

Winter...

1 cup Epsom salt

1 tablespoon baking soda

1/4 teaspoon Cypress Oil

1/4 teaspoon Bay Oil

1/4 teaspoon Eucalyptus Oil

1/2 teaspoon Jasmine Water

4 drops Green food coloring (optional)

Combine all ingredients in a small bowl.

Make sure food coloring is completely absorbed and color is even.

Store in clear glass bottles.

Add roughly 1/4 of mix to running water in bath.

Enough for two baths

words and such...

Mind:

Body:

Soul:

Autumn...

It's that time again, when the leaves change colors, the cold air begins to settle in again, and we wait only days for family and friends gather to us once again and share memories as well as make new ones. For those days, this bath mix is special and your time to yourself is all your own. Remember that during this time of year, your time is in more demand and getting pulled in a thousand directions is the normal day for you. Taking a few minutes for yourself can help keep you on your toes and active in all you do. It's also easy to lose yourself in your tasks and it only takes a few minutes to get back on track. Enjoy the holidays and gathers and meet them with enthusiasm.

Autumn...

1 cup Epsom salt

1 tablespoon baking soda

1/4 teaspoon Clove Oil

1/4 teaspoon Thyme Oil

1/4 teaspoon St. John's Shield Flower Oil

1/2 teaspoon Jasmine Water

Combine all ingredients in a small bowl.

Store in clear glass bottles.

Add roughly 1/4 of mix to running water in bath.

Enough for two baths

words and such...

Mind:

Body:

Soul:

Backyard...

It's that time of year again when most of our time is spent outdoors, at picnics, going to the lake, or a planned barbeque in our own backyards. We love our outdoor endeavors and make big plans for company both expected and unexpected. Prepare for the day with a bath that gets you in the spirit of the season. Along with the grilling, swimming, camping, and cold drinks, there's nothing more relaxing than a bath that prepares you to keep up the pace of being relaxed! So enjoy the season and all it has to offer and don't forget the sunscreen!

Backyard...

1 cup Epsom salt

20 drops Eucalyptus Oil

20 drops Bergamot Oil

20 drops Lemon Oil

1 Tablespoon Rosewater

4 drops Yellow food coloring (optional)

Combine all ingredients in a small bowl.

Make sure food coloring is completely absorbed and color is even.

Store in clear glass bottles.

Add roughly 1/4 of the mix into running water in bath.

Enough for two baths

words and such...

Mind:

Body:

Soul:

Simple times...

Things are running smoothly, everything is on task, and there's nothing left to do but enjoy the time you have to relax and just be. Add a bath to that time and relish in the peace and quite you have worked so hard to accomplish. It's your day now. There are no errands to run, no practice to pick up anyone from, no phone calls to make, or letters to send out. You've finished your work, your giving have given those who are the recipients of your giving quite time, and now, there's nothing more to do than just sit back, and enjoy the time. You've earned it. Begin with a simple bath salt that is not overwhelming or underrated. The mix is just right for a day like this and it's just your kind of day. Doing nothing are the things we desire the most, and now, you can.

Simple times...

1 cup Epsom salt

1 cup Dead Sea salt

1 tablespoon Rosewater or Orange-water

Combine all ingredients in a small bowl.

Store in clear glass bottles.

Add roughly 1/4 of the mix into running water in bath.

Enough for two baths

words and such...

Mind:

Body:

Soul:

Light kind of day...

Some days we have a few things on our to do list, but not that many and they do not require our entire day to finish. This is the sort of day when the world we created for ourselves only asks of a little of our time, and we are ready to answer that call, then take the rest of the day as our own. For days such as this we can prepare for both the tasks that need our attention and the time we have to ourselves. These are easy kind of days, nothing too stressful is occurring, nothing is pressing for our attention, and everything we needed to finish is now complete. Just a light sort of day. So celebrate and enjoy!

Light kind of day...

1 cup Epsom salt

1 tablespoon baking soda

1/4 teaspoon Fig Oil

1/4 teaspoon Peach Oil

1/4 teaspoon Vanilla Oil

1/2 teaspoon Jasmine Water

Combine all ingredients in a small bowl.

Store in clear glass bottles.

Add roughly 1/4 of the mix into running water in bath.

Enough for two baths

words and such...

Mind:

Body:

Soul:

Good feeling...

Sometimes, those gray hairs are not as many as you think they may be. And sometimes, you wake up and just know the day is going to be great. Hold onto that feeling all day by starting it with a special bath. Hold onto that feeling of confidence and charm the entire day and remember that when you are happy, it is likely that those around you will also be happy, making the day even more special than you already knew it would be. There is nothing like having the world on your side and knowing that it is! When you know everything is going your way, you know your going to feel great all day long. The day is yours to take!

Good feeling...

1 Cup Epsom salt

10 drops peppermint oil

15 drops of red food coloring (optional)

1 teaspoon glycerin

Mix all ingredients in a small bowl.

Make sure food coloring is completely absorbed and color is even.

Store in clear glass bottles.

Add small handful to running water in bath.

Enough to make two baths

words and such...

Mind:

Body:

Soul:

www.ingramcontent.com/pod-product-compliance
Lightning Source LLC
Chambersburg PA
CBHW081809280526
45789CB00008B/3068